The Ebb and Flow

Life After Miscarriage

Author's Note

This book is an anthology of poems and reflections written during my miscarriage and in the months to follow as I continue to heal. The poems are raw and at times graphic. The reflections attempt a hopeful optimism, but sometimes fall short. This is not a faith-based devotional, but I do pray my faith is reflected throughout.

My views are my own.

There is not one way to grieve a miscarriage. There is not one way to process how you feel. There is not one right way to conceptualize everything that happens to you or how to manage it. I cannot tell you what is right or wrong. I can only share my experience. These recollections are partly for my catharsis and a tribute to my sweet Shiloh, gone before twelve weeks, and for you, if you have suffered child loss. I do not know your pain, not fully. But I do know you are not alone.

Notable Trigger Warnings: miscarriage, graphic depictions of miscarriage, pregnancy after loss

To Shiloh,

Our second child.

The one we never got to meet.

The one who showed me new depths of love and grief.

"Drink some water, try to relax."
Brown turns to red
As my blood clumps together.
"We'll talk to the provider and then call you back."
Not even an hour passes
Blood pours from my body in one condemning gush
Clump after clump, no choice but to flush
Are you my baby? I wonder, tears running like the blood between my legs.
Shapeless. Lifeless. Loved.
Cramps tear at my insides. Ripping down the walls painstakingly crafted,
snagging the thread of hope I cling to in vain.

"We're going to do everything we can to take care of **you.**"
Don't you mean us? There's two of us here, right? My baby has a chance,
right?
I ask.
The tone changes.
The mood shifts.
"We won't know until the ultrasound."
I can see it on your face. Hear it in your tone.
My body once more will be just that—my own.

Hours pass. The cramps increase.
"Anything for the pain?"
Just Tylenol, please.
It hurts so bad, but I can't risk hurting you.
Not if you're still with me.
Please still be with me.

The cramps claw at my insides, find the hope and rip it free.
I take something stronger.
I wait a while longer.
Was that a heartbeat?
I shouldn't hope.

The walk to the bathroom is slow.
It's when I pull it from me that I know.
That ceramic bowl is cold and unfeeling;
its stark white perfection sullied by the depths of my despair.
How many times have I apologized for bleeding today?
Will that image ever fade?

The doctor says it's not my fault.
Of this he's 100% certain.
Yet I feel culpable.
This body that was supposed to protect you has expelled you.
It ripped you from your home.

"It's your body's way of getting rid of something wrong."
You were a gift.
"Wait two months and try again."
There is no gift exchange.
"Trust me, you wanted a healthy baby. Not one you'd have to take care of
for the rest of its life."
I wanted you, little one. Please know I wanted you.

I wrote the preceding poem the day that I miscarried. There were so
many emotions coursing through me. I learned later that part of this is
because miscarriage triggers a similar—possibly the same—hormonal
discharge as labor. I have never had a strong poker face. Composure is
difficult for me to maintain. With anger, maybe, but rarely sadness,
never grief.

I needed an outlet, but what could I say that hadn't been said already? How many times could I tell my husband I was sad? How many ways could I convey that I was devastated and broken? How could I speak about my pain and agony while my then two-year-old son was playing on the floor—aware but seemingly unaffected by the emotions around him? I turned to writing. To imagery and expression that words alone could not convey. Then I posted it. Maybe it is a vanity of sorts. But I needed this pain to be seen. For as much as I long to not be a burden, I could not bear this alone. But I felt alone. My husband had lost a child. My parents and his had lost a grandchild. But for me it was more than just a loss. My body had become crime scene, victim, and perpetrator.

It was not my fault.

The doctor said that so many times as if it were mantra. I understand, medically, that 1 in 4 pregnancies end this way. I understand, medically, that miscarriage before twelve weeks is indicative of a genetic misalignment, a pregnancy that could not reach fruition in even the best of circumstances. I understand... and yet none of it made sense. It consumed me. A well-meaning individual told me that it did not need to become my personality. It didn't. And yet it did.

I relived those moments, writing them out in an attempt to process.

THE BEGINNING

Brown spots, just a little.
Bright red, just a little more.
A building ache inside my gut.
From deep within I feel it pour.
One plop. Two plops.
Please God, no more.
            That gentle trickle
            Seeping. Creeping.
            The proverbial clock
            Ticking. Ticking.   A sudden gush
                           A frantic rush
                           And the blood came pouring down.

"Breathe, deep breaths, breathe."
Blood soaks my shorts, stains my thigh.
Briefly: *am I going to die?*
Another cramp, another bit of me to cleave.

I don't want to sit down.
I can't bear to stand.
"Here, squeeze my hand."
Deep breaths in, deep breaths out.
"Thompson?"
I let you leave.

"Is someone with you?"
My husband's meeting me.
"Can you tell us what's going on?"
It started yesterday.
I can't stop bleeding.
The cramps started this morning.
I can't stop bleeding.
Then there were these clots.
They were so big. I heard them fall.
"Any tissues?"
Oh no. Oh no no.
I don't want to believe.

Did I flush my baby?
"Does this hurt?"
I can't stop bleeding.
It just aches.
There's no reprieve.

The Ultrasound

Cool jell spreads over my belly.
There's so much pressure,
So much pain.
A faint whooshing sound.
"I'm just going over your ovaries."
I'm just going insane.

I don't want to use the bathroom.
I'm scared of what I'll see.
Luke points out that I'm wearing a
diaper.
We laugh.
Another ultrasound awaits. I really
have to pee.

I stand, wondering how bad.
well
I've soaked through my diaper.
Into my gown.
Onto the pad.

Two new gowns. One front, one back.
A pair of grippy socks
"Down the hall to the left."
I clutch Luke's hand.
Hobble those few steps.
No one bats an eye to see someone so bereft.

With each step I feel the
fresh blood pooling.
No.
I sit, feel it shift.
No.
The last thread of hope
indelicately unspooling.
No.
Involuntarily I tense, as if I
could make it stop.
PLOP

Insult to injury
It didn't slide free.
I have to remove it—*my
baby?*
From me.

It's not over.
Down the hall, we turn right.
Everything's gone wrong.
"As we thought, it's a miscarriage."
On the bed, scoot to the edge
Please don't let this take long.

Feet up, legs wide
That standard discomfort deep inside.
I tremble.
"Does that hurt?"
No, it's okay.
As much as it can be, anyway.

He pulls back.
Blood pours down.
A horror scene behind tented gown.

Again.
Again.
Dear God, please not again.
"I'm having trouble seeing due to the clots."
I'm sorry.
Nurse: "Do you need a cup?"
Doctor: "No, it's just blood."

Just blood.
***Just** blood.*
Just blood.

Cold certainty trickles like the warm blood down my skin.
Your body is gone.
Flushed away.
Never seen again.
I'm sorry.

We had moved two days prior to my miscarriage. The day before the move, I had a horribly stressful day of work. My doctor suggested I had strained myself. I was supposed to take it easy and relax, but then the nightmare began.

It was a horror movie I could not wake from, a crime scene I was living in. There was so much blood. If you have been where I have, I think you know. I do not think you need me to tell you that, but I cannot stop talking about it. Even as I write this paragraph, there are tears in my eyes. After my miscarriage, every single cycle after my miscarriage, I would fear the day the blood would come again. Could I ever trust that it was *just* a period? Will I ever stop being reminded of the way my insides sloughed off inside me, bringing my baby with them?

I can still feel the way the blood poured out. He was a kind doctor. He had humored me in suggesting lighter—baby safe—pain medication even though he had to know that my baby was already gone. He was not cruel, but he became clinical. There is not really a polite way to talk someone through the removal of blood clots for an internal examination I suppose.

My body had become a crime scene. I answered their questions. I walked them through the day. I described my pain.

I was a victim of unfortunate circumstance. An innocent bystander caught up in the pain of a fallen world. I tried not to cry too hard because I did not want to interfere with his examination. I almost *apologized* for the blood clots. As if there was something I could have done to prevent them. The miscarriage was not my fault. I could not control the blood clots.

And yet I still felt a perpetrator. Not for killing my baby, no.

But for abandoning them.

I did not know what was happening to me. I did not know what the blood meant. I did not know that it was tissues. I did not know. But I cannot help but think I should have.

When that final part of me was ripped away, I should have done something.

I should have stumbled to the door and asked Luke to get a nurse.

I should have reached into the toilet and pulled the remnants of my baby, indiscernible from the wreckage of its home from the bowl.

A toilet. Part of my baby was in the toilet. And I flushed.

Will I ever not feel guilty? Can I forgive myself? Nearly a year later and I am still not sure that I have figured it out. It is difficult and messy. But grief always is.

We purchased our house
And made plans for each room.
We labeled one "nursery"
For the baby in my womb.

I wanted fresh paint, a homier look
Always underestimating the time that it took.
"Let's save the kitchen and nursery for last."
Move in day was close, boxes still not packed
Those rooms could wait until the chaos was past.

What is that room now?
What do we do?
Can it be a nursery knowing there'll never be you?
Is it better or worse that it isn't complete?
What might've been a shrine is now a visual of our grief.

We still call it the nursery.
It's as messy as my heart.
Random toys, odds and ends
A whole future dream torn apart.

You'll never come home here.
This won't ever be your space.
But we can't just repurpose.
We can't just replace.

So this room sits untouched
We'll save it for last
Until the ocean of grief is perhaps not so vast.

Our house is coming together.
There's more floor space, less boxes;
More order, less obnoxious.
In the midst of a storm so difficult to weather.

We snuggled on the couch, not yet ready to be awake
Flowers of condolences brighten up our space.
Through the back window the sun shows its face.
I feel something in my heart break.

It's a typical Saturday
There's nothing out of the ordinary
Everything feels the same except the grief I now carry.
I never thought it would be this way.

You were supposed to be here
In seven months or less
Now everything about you is an unanswered guess
Oh how I wish grief could be linear

I wish there was a marker that we could reach and have the pain end
Instead it hides in the background of good times and bad
A new reason to grieve the life I wish you'd had
Another piece of my heart to rend.

There's still goodness to be found
There's still joy to be had,
Even if right now happiness feels bad.
God is still good and his mercies abound.

I was offered a lot of advice from a lot of well-meaning people. Multiple women reached out who had experienced their own loss(es). They gave me suggestions for how to cope.

I did not have any sort of body to bury. I did not have a baby item bought for them yet. I found myself filled with this envy for people who miscarried later in pregnancy. How messed up is that? I was envious that a mom knew she had lost a boy. I was jealous that a mom had a body of sorts to bury. It was not right. It was not fair. But it was grief. Grief is messy and cruel and at times nonsensical.

I longed to have some sort of closure. I was so desperate to know *anything* about who my baby might have been. I was angry that I had not gotten to know anything about them. I was angry that I miscarried at a point that a growing majority of the population does not see as anything "real." I was "hardly" pregnant. I do not know my baby's gender. I was grieving so much and yet somehow feeling that I did not have "enough" to grieve. What does that even mean? I don't know. I know I'd never say it to anyone else in my position, but somewhere in me I felt it. I needed to "make" my baby "real." I needed them to be a person, not just "the baby" or worse "it."

According to Google search, Shiloh can mean tranquil, abundance, and His gift; I was praying for tranquility, for the storm to settle. I was experiencing love and kindness in abundance. This baby was, and is, a gift from God, no matter how short their life with me. And thus, our sweet babe got their name.

Naming Shiloh gave me some level of closure, somehow solidifying them as a person. I am still emotional when my friends refer to them by name when referencing my loss. I was still however left with the question of what to do with their room. Again, I was given lots of well-meant advice for that space. We moved nearly a year after I wrote that poem to move across the state for my husband's new job. In that time, all I had managed to do was shove all of the explicitly baby items into the closet so that I could open the door without wanting to break down. Eventually a few of my son's toys ended up in there but it remained empty. Unfinished.

At first, it felt too soon to do anything to the room. Repurposing felt too much like forgetting. Setting it up as a nursery because we knew we would one day try again felt too much like replacing. Then time went on as time does and it just remained undone. Eventually, we began preparing for a move. I was expecting our third child then and I realized I was actually grateful that I would not have to bring them home to that room, to Shiloh's space. I suppose without realizing it I had allowed the room to become a shrine of sorts. Again, I would never say it to anyone else but to me it felt wrong. I think it would have been particularly challenging for me to use that space—grief and joy raging war on postpartum hormones. I do not know for sure, of course, but I have always been one to linger over the "what ifs" and "maybes." I am grateful I did not have to know.

The problem with the "rainbow baby"
Is it presumes a few things true:
I'm willing to risk the pain again
And there could be a replacement of you.

It's not like an offer on a house;
There's always another to see.
It's not like an insurance claim,
I've not wrecked my car, I've lost my baby.

I know it's said with the best of intentions.
I know it's meant to bring hope.
But it neglects to consider the trauma
And implication's a slippery slope.

This baby was a gift
More precious than a gem
Trials of life may be storms
But the problem was never them.

Lord willing, we'll conceive again
And we'll bring that baby to term
But that gain does not equal our loss
And that reality I want you to affirm.

It's not wrong to talk of the "rainbow baby."
You say it with the best intention.
Yet whether our family grows big or stays small
Sweet Shiloh, will always have a mention.

The "rainbow baby" is a concept that I had always found quite beautiful. The themed maternity and newborn photos were heartwarming and sweet—I was shocked to realize how much I hated it being said to me. It is, perhaps, my least favorite of all well-meant advice that came my way.

I hated this idea that somehow everything would get better or be made right when we would get another child. Partially it angered me because it was not guaranteed. Now, to be clear, having a miscarriage does not mean you are likely to have another. However, it did not mean that I would not, either. That was part of my fear and anxiety with every menstrual cycle. I was so terrified that I would have to live through that grief again.

Then my friend Megan reminded me of the original rainbow. If you are not familiar, the book of Genesis depicts the time that God flooded the world. When the flood ended and the earth dried, God used a rainbow to signify His promise to never again flood the world. Now, this reminder might sound similar to the rainbow baby commentary but there is a distinction: The rainbow at its core is the symbol of God's faithfulness. This means that no matter how many times I am flooded by grief, God is there. There is a plan and purpose in all things. I know that God works all things for good. And, in the midst of all the grief, I could see the good within our loss.

Numerous women reached out to me, thanking me for sharing my story. There was something in hearing about someone else's loss that made them feel less alone. There was something about my ability to openly share that they found healing. Those responses are why I am here writing this now. It has been so painful and hard, but yet there has been good.

I think that is one of the other things that bothers me with the rainbow baby commentary. I know the metaphorical "storm" is the miscarriage itself, not the baby. In my head, though, it is linked. To me it feels like saying the baby was the negative and for me that is the furthest thing from the truth. Shiloh, for the little time we had them, was a gift. A blessing. A precious life gone too soon.

Beyond my frustration with this implication that a new baby would somehow fix my pain or make it all "worth it." I also hated this inherent assumption that we would try again. From some people, this came across in a callous exchange sort of way. One of my ER nurses had an array of colorful commentary that I doubt I will be able to finish this book without reflecting on but one of her throughlines was most certainly: you can just try again for a healthier baby.

Other people, however, were well-meaning and kind. It was no secret that Luke and I desired a large family after all. They were not as lovely as my ER nurse who told me to wait six weeks and try again, but still everyone seemed certain that we would one day try again. It was the big assurance in those first few days or weeks. One person asked me if I wanted to try again. One. It took everything in me not to hug her and sob because for the first moment I felt *seen*. I know everyone was so well-intentioned, but I could not help but feel that they were not pausing to consider my trauma. I could not have a period without hyperventilating.

After having our first child, Jesse, I often reflected on how easy that pregnancy and delivery was for me. I said things like, "if they're all like this, I'll pop out babies for as long as it makes financial sense." Was it my hubris that caused my miscarriage? No. But man some days it felt like it. It took time to heal and to process. I am pregnant now, fourteen weeks and some days, as I type this. I often joke that if anything were to happen to this baby I would need to be committed. The truth is, I do not think it is that much of a joke. At the very least, right now, I think a second miscarriage would be it for me. The idea of experiencing this again... I do not see how I could do it. I admire the strength of the women I know who have miscarried numerous times and dared to try again. You are resilient. I admire the strength of the women who miscarried and chose to never try again. You know and embrace your emotional boundaries and limits.

I do not think I need to justify or further explain exactly how traumatic my miscarriage was for me. But this feels as good a time as any to tell you about the Worst Nurse Ever. Not revealing where I miscarried or the name of the nurse, is the barest kindness I can manage for this woman. From the moment I entered the room, she was horrible.

Picture this: I enter the ER room alone—my boss has gone back to work; my husband has not made it to me yet—and I am hyperventilating. I am sobbing and rapidly breathing. Trying to keep composure even as I feel blood pouring out of me like a horror sequence.

This nurse comes near, and she asks me, "you want a healthy baby, right?"

I sob out a yes and try to calm down, anticipating the beginning of another "calm down, stress isn't good for the baby" speech, like my former boss had given me on the way over.

But instead, she told me to wait two months and try again. She told me that this was my body's way of getting rid of something that was wrong. She said to me, "you want a healthy baby. Not one that is sick or needs taken care of the rest of their life."

At the end of her advice, she told me that I was "too hormonal to want to hear any of it right now."

Listen, I know that I am a prolife Christian.

I know not everyone would recognize that baby as a life.

But I think EVERYONE can file those things under "things you don't say to the weeping woman still *clearly* hoping her baby is somehow alive."

Months later—nearly a full year later—I am still filled with rage at this woman and the things she said to me. Particularly her parting line when it was all said and done.

I am lying there, and I am still bleeding. In the haze of my grief, I am beginning to wonder at what point miscarriage becomes medical emergency. How much blood can I lose? Is this normal? I ask and the doctor, the kind doctor, told me it was typical.

"The body has ways of taking care of this kind of thing. It is kind of cool how it can do that," says The Worst Nurse Ever.

Kind. Of. Cool.

Is it cool to be the Final Girl in your real-life horror film?

I can barely muster *gratefulness* for not having needed a D&C procedure. Perhaps I have not healed enough.

Or perhaps we should add that to the list.

Despite experiencing miscarriage, that woman had no idea how to talk about it. Sometimes I do not either. It is at times absurdly hard to acknowledge Shiloh. All of that mental work to personify them and make them more real to me, all of that desire for them to be acknowledged, the fear of them being forgotten, and sometimes I just cannot do it.

Miscarriage is a bummer topic. There is not a value judgment on that. It just... is. Unfortunately, it is one you have to navigate—particularly if you are married. People just love to ask about children. Before we had our first child, people wanted to know when we were going to start having children. I still do not think that there is anything *wrong* with that line of questioning, even now. People are by nature curious. People love to share.

I just wish we all universally recognized that it is a *loaded* question. Infertility, miscarriage, child loss—you are inviting those possible answers when you ask that question. You are potentially putting someone in the position where they have to decide if they want to divulge. It is hard sometimes.

We already have one son here on earth and it invites its own set of questions such as: "Do you have any other children?" or "So when are you giving Jesse a sibling?"

In a perfect world, I would answer that I have three children: a child on earth, one in heaven, and expecting a third. In a perfect world, I would say, "he has one sibling in heaven, now, and another due in January."

But I am not perfect. Far too often I allow concern for the other person's comfort—and fear that I will need to justify myself—to dictate how I answer.

I suppose in truth there is no real "perfect," but I wish that I would be braver and face that loaded question head on. I wish that I would always, boldly, proclaim Shiloh's existence. They were here. They mattered. They still matter.

I am Shaniah. I am a mom of three. One boy, one in heaven, and one in my belly. That is who I am. Social convention should not take that from me. Do not let it take it from you.

September 18, 2023: A perfect world

Shoulda
"You said you have children? How many?"
Two, but I miscarried one.
"Oh, I'm so sorry."
Thank you. Jesse, he's our son.
"How old is he?"
Two and a half.
"Oh, that's nice. And the other…?"
I was twelve weeks. We didn't know.
But… we call them Shiloh.
"Such a lovely name."

Coulda
"You have children? How many?"
Two, but one miscarried.
…
Jesse, my son, he's two and a half.
"Oh, that's nice."
…
They were supposed to share a birthday.
…
We named them Shiloh.
…
How about you?

Didn't.
"You said you have children? How many?"
Say it.
I have a son, Jesse.
Say it.
"How old is he?"
Say it.
Two and a half.
"Oh, that's nice."
Say it.
How about you?
Coward.

Eventually life settles. I am not sure if grief gets smaller or if the capacity to bear it simply increases but somehow you find time has *passed* and it wasn't always painful. Directly following the loss of Shiloh, I left my old job and found a new one. It was a healthier work environment. I was happier. Jesse was thriving. My husband had started a new job as well. Life moved on. Days turned to weeks turned to months.

There were moments when the grief resurfaced. Again, I would be reminded every month of my loss as a new cycle began. To make it worse, my cycle became very irregular. I had once been so predictable that I knew I was pregnant with Jesse the day before I expected my period. Now I had no idea when the blood would come. Or how much there would be. Sometimes it took so long that I would take a pregnancy test. Then I would analyze the blood in the toilet or on the pad wondering if it was *just* blood. I used to use a combination of pads and tampons based on flow and comfort. Now I almost *needed* tampons to limit how much blood flow I would have to see or feel. Despite an anxiety attack about once a month, life moved on. Shiloh was not a daily thought. Then February came. My due date was Jesse's birthday.

When I had first done those calculations, I had felt guilty. I worried that his birthday would be overshadowed by a newborn or subpar due to his heavily pregnant mother. Instead, I experienced one of the most bittersweet days of my life.

Grief and joy dance hand in hand
Theirs is the song of life.
Sorrow, pain, and amazing grace
Bright light in times of strife

Yesterday, the third year of our son
But also, the day we should have met,
our yet unknown little one.
The grief it comes in waves.

Those early months it crushed me.
Sent me swirling in its grasp.
These days it laps at the shore
errant high waves draw a gasp.

That cold dousing of reality
The reminder of your loss
I keep my eyes to the horizon
Defy the albatross.

Each storm begets a rainbow.
My savior has walked this
tempestuous sea.
One day we'll meet you, Shiloh
'Til then in his arms you'll be.

In May 2024 I learned I was expecting. It was not just a late period. It was three pregnancy tests worth of confirmations. If grief was a tidal wave, anxiety became a tsunami. I called my doctor immediately to let them know. Apparently, they do not schedule the first prenatal visit until you are ten weeks pregnant.

I am not sure if that's common practice or not. When I was pregnant with Jesse, they saw me immediately. When I was pregnant with Shiloh, there was a staffing issue in the office and so I was not scheduled for a visit until much later—in fact, I hadn't even been seen before I miscarried.

However, it usually works, I had basically a bit over a month to wait to know if my pregnancy was "real." I needed a doctor to look at me and tell me I was really pregnant. I needed to know medically that I was okay. I immediately started following all of the pregnancy protocols. No medicine aside from my thyroid medicine. I called my PCP to ask for bloodwork because I remembered it needed to be checked once a trimester. This had been missed with Jesse and he came out fine—but nothing was to be left to chance this time.

I also began experiencing the worst of pregnancy symptoms. I was nauseous if I did not eat. Nauseous if I ate the wrong things. I was chronically tired. I was constipated. I was the worst of pregnancy.

I stored up every negative like it was piles of gold. These symptoms confirmed my pregnancy. The baby was real. The hormones were there, present, and strong, and so my baby must be too. Of course, that made good days really difficult. I could not enjoy the reprieve from pregnancy symptoms because it might mean the hormones were gone—not settled, not acclimated—gone.

It was a lot. I was not the poster child of Christian trust or faith. I was a desperate woman trying to lean on her own power. It was all I talked about or focused on. It did not help that we were prepping to move. If you will recall, we moved two days before my miscarriage. I knew I had not caused my miscarriage. But what if I had? I lived in this constant tension between wanting and needing to contribute at work and home but needing to rest and all the while being terrified of triggering loss.

It had been a while since I experienced a healthy pregnancy. I could not remember what it all had felt like. I was second-guessing pains along my abdomen. I was worried about how tired I was. Extra discharge is normal in that first trimester, but I needed to go to the bathroom every time I felt it just to make sure; I do not know what I would have done if I had experienced spotting. I think God knew I could not take it.

Anxiously, the days passed, and I made it to my first prenatal visit.

I'm in a room alone again
Laid bare but for that gown
Anxiety grinds patience thin
Each time I shove it down.

A standard visit, just a prenatal check
No signs of anything amiss
And yet I'm still a nervous wreck.
No more ignorance, no bliss

Am I truly pregnant?
Does that little life still grow?
Trauma leaves a bitter remnant
No true peace until I know.

The doctor is kind
She listens, she cares
An ultrasound to ease my mind
See there? There's...

Crying. Weeping.
I see my baby
They're alive not sleeping.
A beating heart—for sure not maybe

And then I hear it,
that sweet swift sound
My worries I forget
As joyous tears abound.

I do not have words for the absolute love and adoration I have for my doctor that day. She was the antithesis to the Worst Nurse Ever. It was my first time meeting her and I am genuinely sad that I had to leave the practice since we moved. At the first prenatal visit, they listen for baby's heartbeat. I told her of my anxieties, and she warned me that it would be a 50/50 chance of hearing the baby.

This is not because something is wrong, but simply because they are so small and competing with much louder noises. I still wanted her to try, but she could see the worry. She offered to do a bedside ultrasound to try and see the baby first. If we could ascertain the location, it would be easier to hear.

I was so scared, but then there was my baby. My sweet, sweet, tiny baby and the tiny flutter of their heartbeat. I wept. Then she used the doppler and I cried again. My baby was there, really there, and their heart was beating. A week or two later I saw them again in the size and dating ultrasound. Still there. Still beating. Still growing. No abnormalities.

Life Now

The anxiety is not gone, not fully. I still worry about what I do. I still long to start showing. My pants are tighter, certainly, but there is no proper bump yet. I know it is early. I just long for every physical milestone, every tangible bit of proof that my baby is still here.

I know I need to trust God. I think that I do. My issue is truly just that I do not know His plan. Maybe there is more loss for me to experience. I do not know if that's pessimism or realism, but either way it is how I feel. I am not leaning into the trust that God will preserve this pregnancy. I am leaning into the trust that—whatever happens—God will continue to provide for me. I hope, I pray, I anxiously yearn for His will to be that this baby reach full term and enter this world alive and well.

But I just do not know. That is why they call it faith, I suppose.

In a way, this feels like a bad time to write this book. Journal? I'm still not sure what I'd call it. I haven't made it through my third pregnancy yet. There's so much more "life after miscarriage" to experience, but it felt important to do this now. We are coming up on the one-year anniversary of my miscarriage. It is nearly Shiloh's birthday.

I am not sure if that's strange or not. My dear friend gave me a necklace featuring two amethyst stones for my February babies. I love it for its sentiment. It is so special to me how she continues to remember and allow me to grieve for Shiloh so many months after the fact. She never makes me feel like the time for grieving has passed. This was a bitterness for me when my church removed me from their prayer list. Obviously, I don't think my miscarriage should have been on there forever, but something in me said, "oh, you think it's been long enough" when I saw it was taken off. But I digress.

Shiloh's due date is significant to me. But so is July 25. My son was born two weeks early and we celebrate that day as his birthdate. For better or worse, Shiloh entered this world on July 25. I wanted to write this and publish it as a tribute to them on their first heavenly birthday. Their short life changed mine irrevocably. They are forever part of my story, forever in my heart.

I pray that one day in heaven, I will get to hold them in my arms.